A COMPREHENSION OF ALLERGIC RHINITIS

A Comprehensive Guide to the Understanding, Treatment, and Recovery from Allergic Rhinitis

CARL JUAN

Table of Contents

Introductory

As a medical disorder, allergic rhinitis causes nasal passage irritation in response to allergens in the air. Common allergens that can provoke allergic rhinitis include pollen, dust mites, pet dander, and mold spores. The immune system of a person with allergic rhinitis responds to these allergens by generating substances like histamine, which causes symptoms including:

• Sneezing

• Congested or runny nose

• Dry or itchy eyes

- Throat or ear itching

- Coughing

- Fatigue

These symptoms are often seasonal when induced by outdoor allergens like pollen, or perennial (year-round) when caused by interior allergens such dust mites or pet dander. Allergic rhinitis can dramatically damage a person's quality of life, leading to discomfort, sleep problems, and reduced everyday functioning.

The most common forms of allergic rhinitis are:

1. For example, hay fever in the spring or allergies to grass and tree pollen in the fall are examples of seasonal allergic rhinitis.

2. Allergens found inside the home, such as dust mites, mold, pet dander, and cockroach allergens, are common causes of the year-round condition known as perennial allergic rhinitis.

Avoiding allergens is the first line of defense against allergic rhinitis, but there are other ways to treat the condition, such as using antihistamines, decongestants, nasal corticosteroid sprays, and allergy needles. It's best to see a doctor if you think you have allergic rhinitis so that you may get a proper diagnosis and advice on the best course of therapy.

CHAPTER ONE
Allergic Rhinitis: Classification and Types

Duration and specific allergens can be used to categorize allergic rhinitis into distinct subtypes. The two main categories are defined by how long symptoms last and how quickly they appear:

1. Allergic Rhinitis during the Seasons (SAR):

• Allergies to pollen, grass, or mold are another name for hay fever.

Occurs in the spring (tree pollen), summer (grass pollen), and fall (weed pollen), when those allergens are at their peak.

• Outdoor allergens are a common cause of symptoms.

Tree pollen, grass pollen, and plant pollen are common allergies.

2. Allergy that lasts for more than a year:

• Indoor allergens are often the cause, thus symptoms can last all year long.

• It's possible for symptoms to last all year.

Dust mites, mold spores, animal fur, and cockroach allergies are just a few of the most common allergens found inside.

Classification of allergic rhinitis is also possible according to the severity and duration of symptoms:

1. Rhinitis Allergic, Intermittent:

• fewer than four days per week or fewer than four weeks per year of symptoms.

2.Allergic Rhinitis That Won't Go Away:

• Symptoms persist for more than four weeks per year, or four days per week.

In addition, the immunological systems underpinning allergic rhinitis allow for the following classifications:

1. Allergic Rhinitis Caused by IgE:

- Allergenic rhinitis is the most prevalent form of the condition.

Immunoglobulin E (IgE) antibodies are at the heart of the allergic reaction that defines this condition.

- Common allergy symptoms result from the release of IgE antibodies and histamine in response to exposure to allergens.

2. Allergic Rhinitis Not Caused by Immunoglobulin E

- IgE antibodies are not a primary driver of this form of rhinitis.

- It is less prevalent and may not be helped by the typical antihistamines used to treat allergies.

- Some individuals may suffer symptoms due to different immunological mechanisms or sensitivities to irritants, such as smoke or pollution.

3. Allergic Rhinitis with a Twist

• It's possible for people to have reactions that are both IgE-mediated and non-IgE-mediated.

It's crucial to note that allergic rhinitis can vary in severity and individual triggers, and the classification may help guide therapy and management techniques. Consultation with a healthcare provider or allergist is recommended for accurate diagnosis of allergic rhinitis and selection of the most appropriate treatment.

Allergens and Common Triggers

Allergens, substances that produce an overreaction of the immune system in people who are allergic to them, are widespread. Allergens and their associated common triggers include:

1. Pollen:

• Originating in the flora of the earth. It's a common allergen that sets off symptoms of hay fever in the spring and summer.

2. Microorganisms that call dust, pillows, and sofa cushions home.

3. Messy Pet Hair:

• Animal dander, dander from cats and dogs, and allergens in their fur and feathers.

4. Mould Particles:

• Common in both indoor and outdoor settings with high moisture content.

5. Allergens from Cockroaches:

• Some people, especially those living in cities, may be sensitive to this compound, which has been found in the droppings and saliva of cockroaches.

6. Venomous Insects:

• Bees, wasps, hornets, and fire ants are just some of the insects whose stings or bites might trigger an allergic reaction in some people.

7. The Problem with Food Allergens:

• Common food allergens include peanuts, tree nuts, milk, eggs, soy, wheat, fish, and shellfish.

8. Latex:

• Allergies to natural rubber latex are common among people who work with latex on a regular basis, such as medical personnel.

9. Medications:

• Some people have an adverse reaction to common drugs like penicillin.

10. Sensitizers for the Lungs:

• Irritants like smoke, strong scents, or air pollution may cause non-allergic rhinitis in certain people.

11. Allergens in the Workplace:

• Chemicals, dust, and fumes found in the workplace might trigger allergic reactions in some workers.

12. Allergies to stings from bees, wasps, hornets, and fire ants can be life-threatening.

13. Metals:

• Contact with jewelry made of certain metals, particularly nickel, can trigger skin sensitivities.

14. Products for the Beauty and Hygiene of the Body:

• Cosmetics, lotions, shampoos, and soaps can cause skin allergies in some people because of the ingredients used to make them.

Allergens and triggers, as well as the intensity of allergic reactions, might differ from one person to the next. The severity of an allergic reaction can vary widely, from moderate irritation to life-threatening anaphylaxis. Seek medical attention if you have any reason to believe you have allergies or have ever experienced a severe allergic reaction, and always carry any recommended drugs, such as epinephrine, in case an emergency calls for their use. An allergist can aid in the diagnosis of allergies and offer advice on how best to manage and treat them.

CHAPTER TWO
Identifying Allergic Rhinitis Symptoms

Allergic rhinitis (hay fever) symptoms should be recognized for accurate diagnosis and treatment. The nasal passages are frequently affected by the symptoms of allergic rhinitis, which can range in intensity.

1. **Sneezing:** Frequent and repetitive sneezing is a defining symptom of allergic rhinitis. Allergens are a common cause of this condition.

2."Drippy" or "runny" noses are common symptoms of allergic

rhinitis, which is characterized by a clear, watery discharge from the nose.

3. Nasal congestion occurs when nasal tissues become inflamed and swollen, causing a stuffy sensation.

4. Common symptoms of allergic rhinitis include a burning sensation in the nose, throat, and sometimes the ears. The itchiness is annoying at best.

5. Red, watery eyes are a common symptom of allergic rhinitis, which frequently occurs in tandem with allergic conjunctivitis.

6. Allergic rhinitis symptoms can include a persistent cough that is commonly brought on by postnasal drip.

7. Exhaustion: Allergic rhinitis can contribute to exhaustion and an overall feeling of being poorly, especially when symptoms are strong or prolonged.

8. Allergic rhinitis can cause nasal congestion and inflammation, which can lessen your ability to smell.

9. Ear symptoms such as fullness, popping, or pain may indicate a problem with the Eustachian tube.

10. Headache: Some patients with allergic rhinitis develop headaches, often owing to sinus pressure and congestion.

It's worth stressing that the severity and duration of these symptoms might vary greatly from person to person. Depending on the allergens that cause your symptoms, your seasonal allergic rhinitis could come and go with the seasons. For chronic allergic rhinitis, symptoms can remain throughout the year, often owing to indoor allergens such dust mites, pet dander, or mold.

A doctor or allergist can provide a definitive diagnosis of allergic rhinitis and advise you on the best course of therapy if you are suffering any of the aforementioned symptoms. In extreme situations, allergen-specific immunotherapy (allergy shots) may be necessary in addition to avoidance measures, OTC medications, and prescription drugs.

Alternative Treatments

Allergic rhinitis (also known as hay fever) therapy goals include symptom alleviation, inflammation reduction, and enhancement of patient well-being. The degree of symptoms, the allergens involved, and the patient's personal preferences all play a role in determining the best course of treatment. Common methods for relieving allergic rhinitis include:

1. Avoiding Allergens:

• Avoiding the allergens that cause your symptoms should be your first line of protection. If you have an allergy to pet dander, you may want to keep pets out of the bedroom and use an air purifier, as well as wash bedding and curtains frequently.

2. Medicines available without a prescription:

• Common over-the-counter medications for allergies include antihistamines (like cetirizine and loratadine), decongestants (like pseudoephedrine), and nasal corticosteroid sprays (like fluticasone and budesonide). Nasal corticosteroids can reduce inflammation, while antihistamines alleviate itching, sneezing, and runny nose. For temporary alleviation of nasal congestion, decongestants may be used, but their usage should be monitored closely due to the risk of adverse effects.

3. FDA-Approved Prescription Drugs:

• If OTC drugs are insufficient, your healthcare practitioner may prescribe stronger antihistamines, nasal corticosteroids, or additional medications such leukotriene modifiers (e.g., montelukast) or nasal antihistamines.

4. Sprays for Nasal Congestion Relief:

• Quick relief from nasal congestion can be found with the use of nasal decongestant sprays (such as oxymetazoline), but their usage should be limited to no more than three to four days at a time to prevent the development of a rebound effect.

5. Allergy Shots, or Immunotherapy:

• In order to develop tolerance to allergens, allergen-specific immunotherapy—also known as allergy shots—can be used over the course of several years. Those with severe allergies may find it helpful, as it may give them with prolonged relief.

6. Intranasal Immunotherapy (IVIG):

• As an alternative to allergy injections, sublingual immunotherapy (SLIT) involves administering allergen extracts sublingually. It's an alternative to needles for people who are allergic to specific substances.

7. Irrigating the Nose:

• Using saline nasal sprays or a neti pot can help flush irritants from the nasal passages and lessen symptoms.

8. Natural and Homeopathic Treatments:

- It's not always supported by scientific evidence, but some people get relief from their symptoms by using homeopathic treatments or natural supplements like butterbur, quercetin, or probiotics. Before utilizing any alternative medicine, it's best to talk to a doctor.

9. Surgery: In rare circumstances, when other therapies are inadequate, surgery such as turbinate reduction or septoplasty may be performed to enhance nasal airflow.

Considerations such as the intensity of your symptoms, the allergens implicated, and any preexisting health concerns should inform your treatment decision. If you suffer from allergic rhinitis, you should talk to a doctor or allergist about the best course of action to take. Additionally, it may be important to schedule periodic follow-up sessions so that your progress may be tracked and your therapy can be modified accordingly.

CHAPTER THREE
What It's Like to Have Allergic Rhinitis

Allergic rhinitis (hay fever) is a common ailment that can be difficult to live with, but it is manageable. Some methods for coping with allergic rhinitis are presented below.

1. Learn What Sets you Off by tracking down the allergens that cause your symptoms. As a result, you'll be able to take more precise steps to limit your contact with the allergens in question. Allergens such as pollen, dust mites, pet dander, and mold are frequently encountered.

2. Avoiding Allergens:

• Use allergen-proof pillow and mattress coverings, wash bedding on a regular basis in hot water, and invest in an air purifier with a HEPA filter to make your house more allergy-friendly.

• During peak pollen times, keep windows shut to keep allergens outside where they belong.

Keep pets out of bedrooms and install high-efficiency particulate air (HEPA) filters in your home's heating and cooling systems to reduce your exposure to indoor allergens such pet dander.

Mold growth can be prevented by using a dehumidifier in wet spaces.

3. Consult a medical expert and work out a prescription schedule that works for you. This may include OTC or prescription antihistamines, nasal corticosteroid sprays, or other allergy drugs to ease symptoms.

• Always follow your doctor's orders when taking medication. It may take many days for nasal corticosteroid sprays, in particular, to reach maximum efficacy.

4. Allergy Shots, or Immunotherapy:

• Consider allergen-specific immunotherapy (allergy shots) if your allergic rhinitis is severe and not well-controlled by medicines. You can get long-term relief from your allergies by desensitizing your immune system with allergy shots.

5. Intranasal Immunotherapy (IVIG):

• Sublingual immunotherapy, or allergy drops placed under the tongue, may be an option worth exploring with your healthcare physician.

6. Irrigating the Nose:

• Use saline nasal sprays or a neti pot to clear your nasal passages of allergies and excess mucus.

7. Keep an eye on local pollen counts, and especially on days with high pollen concentrations, try to limit outside activity.

8. Carefully plot your outdoor adventures:

• If you must go outside during peak pollen times, shield your eyes and face with sunglasses and a wide-brimmed hat.

Pollen can be removed from your hair and clothes by taking a shower and changing after spending time outside.

9. Keep your mucous membranes wet by drinking plenty of water; this may help ease some of your symptoms.

10. Be Aware of Your Triggers: Recognize the situations that tend to set off negative reactions in you and work to eliminate them. If you have a food allergy, for instance, you should be very careful to read labels and avoid foods that contain your allergens.

11. Work with an allergist who can correctly diagnose your condition, create a tailored treatment plan, and advise you on how to live with your allergies.

12. Stay Informed: Keep up to date with the latest research and treatments for allergic rhinitis, as new therapies and drugs may become available.

It's important to keep in mind that treating allergic rhinitis is an ongoing process, and it could take some time before you find the approach that works best for you. You can lessen the effect that allergic rhinitis has on your life and improve your quality of life with the appropriate strategy and direction.

Problems and Associated Disorders

Allergic rhinitis (hay fever) is typically considered a relatively benign disorder, but it can develop to numerous consequences and may coexist with other medical conditions. Possible side effects and comorbidities of allergic rhinitis include the following:

Complications:

1. Symptoms of sinusitis include facial pain, pressure, and a thick nasal discharge, and can develop after a bout of allergic rhinitis. Untreated allergic rhinitis can lead to recurring episodes of chronic sinusitis.

2. Nasal polyps: Nasal polyps can form after repeated inflammation and irritation of the nasal passages. Nasal polyps are benign growths that can block airflow and cause a person to lose their sense of smell in the nose or sinuses.

3. Otitis media with effusion (fluid buildup behind the eardrum) and ear infections are two ear issues that allergic rhinitis can aggravate.

4. Symptoms of allergic rhinitis, such as sneezing and nasal congestion, can cause sleep disruptions, which in turn can lead to weariness and worse daily performance.

Concomitant Ailments:

1. People who suffer from both allergic rhinitis and asthma are not uncommon. In some cases, treating allergic rhinitis might help bring asthma under better control.

2. Eczema (atopic): Asthma and eczema together make up what is called the "atopic triad," which also includes allergic rhinitis. There may be a genetic link between these illnesses, which explains why they tend to develop together.

3. People who suffer from allergic rhinitis are more likely to also have food allergies, and the same allergens (such as those connected to pollen) can sometimes cause a reaction when consumed together.

4. Allergic conjunctivitis, which causes the eyes to be itchy and watery, frequently occurs alongside allergic rhinitis.

5. People who suffer from allergic rhinitis may be at a higher risk of developing chronic rhinosinusitis, a disorder characterized by persistent inflammation of the sinuses.

6. In addition to allergic rhinitis, some people have nonallergic rhinitis when exposed to irritants like smoking, strong scents, or shifts in temperature and humidity.

These potential consequences and coexisting diseases should be taken seriously because of the impact they can have on an individual's health and quality of life. In order to effectively manage your allergic rhinitis, handle any difficulties, and receive the best treatment and guidance, it is crucial to collaborate with healthcare professionals including allergists and otolaryngologists. Effective management can lessen the likelihood of problems and boost general health.

Conclusion

Inflammation of the nasal passages caused by an allergic reaction to airborne allergens characterizes allergic rhinitis, more often known as hay fever. Sneezing, a stuffy or runny nose, itchy eyes and throat, coughing, and exhaustion are just some of the annoying side effects of this illness. Seasonal and perennial forms of allergic rhinitis exist, as do milder and more severe forms with diverse immunological causes.

- Allergen avoidance, OTC or prescription drugs, allergen-specific immunotherapy (allergy injections), and behavioral changes are all part of the management of allergic rhinitis. It's crucial to engage with healthcare professionals or allergists to build a comprehensive treatment strategy tailored to your individual situation.

• The quality of life for those who suffer from allergic rhinitis can be greatly enhanced through the identification of triggers, the reduction of allergen exposure, and the observance of a well-designed treatment plan. Better management and preventative interventions are possible when probable consequences and concomitant disorders related to allergic rhinitis are known.

Seek medical help for a proper diagnosis and treatment if you think you might have allergic rhinitis. Allergic rhinitis is a common condition, but with treatment, many people can find relief and lead normal lives again.

THE END